Intermittent Fasting

Burn Fat Extra Fast, Gain Muscle
And Live Longer, Healthier Living

Introduction

I want to thank you and congratulate you for downloading the book, *"Healthy Intermittent Fasting"*.

This book has actionable information on how to use intermittent fasting to lose weight, attain optimal health and obtain many other benefits.

Mankind has been fasting for centuries and throughout history. Sometimes, the fasting wasn't exactly a voluntary activity. Think about it; back in the days, in the hunter gatherer communities, mankind could go for long hours or probably days without food.

Fast forward to the time when man started having organized religion. Fasting is a religious activity that has been in practice for thousands of years; many religious organizations or groups such as the Christians, Muslims and even the Jewish incorporate fasting as part of their religious activities. For instance, it is not surprising to see a Muslim going on 40 days fast in preparation for the Ramadan.

While fasting has, for a long time, been associated with the lack of food and religion, the practice of fasting is now taking a different direction. People are now fasting for a different reason. For instance, in recent times, fasting now supersedes a religious activity. It has come to be known as a health boosting activity. So what's the difference between that and starving for days without food as we see happening in some poverty stricken parts of the world? Well, the difference is that there is a way of fasting that makes you attain these benefits; you just don't go without food for days then expect to be healthy! So how do you go about fasting in a good way to obtain the different benefits?

The most popular type of fasting that serves as a boost to health is known as the intermittent fasting. This book will serve as a master guide on how to achieve optimal health with intermittent fasting. It will cover various aspects of intermittent fasting such as the clear definition of the term intermittent fasting, health benefits and challenges associated with intermittent fasting, methods of intermittent fasting and tips on how to make your fasting very effective. After reading this book, you should be able to incorporate intermittent fasting as part of your everyday lifestyle and boost your health.

Thanks again for downloading this book, I hope you enjoy it!

Table of Contents

Before we can get to the point of discussing the ins and outs of intermittent fasting, let's first understand what intermittent fasting is.

What Is Intermittent Fasting?

While growing up, you may have been told that you require at least three meals especially your breakfast to live a healthy life. On the contrary, recent research has discovered that you do your body more good by skipping some meals. That's where the concept of intermittent fasting comes in. In its simplest terms, intermittent fasting is a type of fasting that requires you to take a break from eating. It is a conscious decision to skip certain meals. In this case, you have to eat, stop, and eat again. In other words, intermittent fasting (commonly referred to as IF) is not really a diet. Instead, it is an eating pattern or a way of scheduling meals in a way that ensures that you get the most out of them. IF does not really change what you eat. Instead, it only changes when you actually eat. When you fast and feast when you want, IF will mean eating calories during a certain window of the day then choosing not to it during the rest of the time.

Additionally, it isn't all crazy about cutting your calories or being obsessed about reading labels (although it definitely does help). In fact, when starting out, you just maintain your calories intake at the level that you are used to. And when you do that, you can be sure that you will derive all the benefits that come with IF (including losing weight, maintaining muscle mass and getting lean). When you start your journey through intermittent fasting, you will soon realize that it is simple enough that you will actually do it but pretty meaningful enough that you will actually notice a difference in your life.

So how does it work?

For us to understand how IF works, it is necessary that we start by learning the difference between the fasted and fed state. When we eat, the body goes into a fed state whereby it is digesting and absorbing food. The fed state starts when you start eating and lasts for up to 3-5 hours when your body digests and absorbs the food that you just ate. At the fed state, it is very hard for the body to burn fat especially because your insulin levels are quite high (when you eat food, insulin is produced in response to trigger the body cells to start absorbing the food from the bloodstream). At that time, the body's #1 priority is to use up the nutrients (mainly glucose) in your bloodstream. But as time goes on, the body then goes into a post-absorptive state- a fancy way of saying that the body is not processing food. This state lasts for about 8-12 hours after your last meal after which your body then goes into the fasted state. When your body is in the fasted state, it is likely to burn more fat because your insulin levels are quite low. At this state, your body can burn the fat that wasn't accessible during your fed state. Unfortunately, given that it takes about 12 hours after our last meal for our bodies to get into the fasted state, it is very rare for our bodies to get into this state. That's why many of us who start IF will lose fat pretty fast without even changing what we've been eating, how much you eat and how often you exercise. This is because fasting essentially puts your body into a fat burning state, which you rarely make it to during your normal eating schedule.

Tip: By cutting out an entire meal, you are highly likely to eat more food in your other meals but still consume a significant caloric deficit (which is very important if you want to lose weight).

Note: The period that you eat your meals is called the window period. During this period, you get to eat as much food as you need and after the window period, you resume fasting. The type of intermittent fasting that you embark on will determine the number of hours for your window period. I will discuss more on that when I mention the methods of intermittent fasting. What's important for now is to keep in mind that your fasting period should last for up to 14 hours straight for your body to enter strict fasting mode.

I know you have many questions to ask about intermittent fasting such as:

- ✓ "Wouldn't my body break down my muscles during the fasting process?"

- ✓ "Is there any science that backs intermittent fasting?"

- ✓ "Isn't it unhealthy to go for that long without food?"

- ✓ "What if I get very hungry during my fasting period?"

- ✓ "Is there any danger to it?"

- ✓ Am I fit for intermittent fasting?"

There is no need to worry a lot. You will get answers to all your questions as you read the book. Let us take it a step further by examining some of the health benefits you stand to derive from intermittent fasting.

Health Benefits Of Intermittent Fasting:

Are there some health benefits you stand to gain from intermittent fasting? Yes, there are a whole lot of health benefits, which your body derives when you follow intermittent fasting. We will discuss some of them in this section.

It Helps In Weight Loss

If you have been looking for a not so stressful method to lose those excess fats in your body, then you have to start considering intermittent fasting to help you lose weight. So how does intermittent fasting help in weight loss?

Whenever you eat your meal, especially carbohydrates/sugar, your body breaks it down to glucose, which is absorbed into the blood stream as blood sugar. In response, the hormone called insulin, which is produced in the pancreas is released into the bloodstream. The role of the insulin is to activate the body cells to absorb the sugar or glucose in the blood for metabolism and storage. When your body secretes insulin, your cells open up to take up the blood glucose.

The body cells carry the glucose to other parts of the body where it is used as energy. In essence, the more sensitive your body is to insulin, the higher the likelihood that you will use the food that you consume efficiently, which will ultimately lead to muscle creation and weight loss.

Some of the glucose/sugar is stored in the liver and within the muscle cells in the form of glycogen. Your glycogen (a form of starch that is stored in you liver and muscles that your body can burn whenever necessary) is however depleted whenever you fast (e.g. while sleeping) and will even be depleted the more when you exercise thus increasing your insulin sensitivity. As such, the meal that follows your workout is stored efficiently (especially as glycogen for muscle cells, which is burned immediately to help you with the recovery process with very little of it being stored as fat).

When you have too much insulin (due to consistently high levels of glucose in your bloodstream), your glycogen stores will probably be full all the time while your bloodstream will probably have enough glucose for your daily calorie requirement as well as surpluses that could be stored as fat. The excess glucose is stored as fats under the skin especially around the abdominal region, thighs and under the arms (subcutaneous fat). Some of the excess glucose is also stored around major organs (visceral fat). As this process continues uncontrollably, you are likely to become overweight or obese.

Intermittent fasting helps you lose weight through various ways:

✓ First, when you stop eating because of the fasting, your body will be stripped of its main source of energy, which is food. Since your body requires energy to function well, it will look for an alternative means to generate this energy. In a bid to survive, your body starts to make use of glycogen stored up in your liver. This process is triggered if you don't eat for 8 hours. After using up the glucose in the liver, if there is no immediate source of energy for the body, it begins to burn or use up the fats stored up inside your body. This process of using up stored up fats by the body to produce energy is called ketosis and this helps you lose weight. The less the amount of blood sugar in your bloodstream, the more fat you burn and the faster you lose weight. The good thing about this process is that your muscles remain untouched while the fats are used up. Just imagine how much more fat you could lose if you combine IF with exercise and a weight loss diet.

Keep the following in mind:

- You lose fat fast when you eat less while on your weight loss diet

- You lose fat fast without exercise and diet when you fast for up to 14-20 hours a day

- You lose fat fast whenever you exercise and if you ensure this exercise is scheduled when you are on a fast

- You burn fat faster because your blood sugar levels are significantly lower since this forces your body to burn lots of more fat for energy while working out.

✓ Secondly, you take in fewer calories when you engage in intermittent fasting and this can lead to long-term weight loss. I mentioned this earlier; while you may eat more food during your feeding time, you are unlikely to eat as much food as you would if you ate several meals, which essentially means that creating a caloric deficit is easy.

✓ The third way that intermittent fasting helps you lose weight is that it helps your body trigger the release a high level of noradrenalin, which is a hormone that helps to breakdown body fats to produce energy for your body. Why does that happen? Well, when your glucose or energy levels are low, the body responds by releasing adrenalin or norepinephrine, which triggers your body to start demanding more energy to keep you alert. Since you don't have ready glucose supplies, your body then responds by pushing the body to burn stored fats for energy (this is the fat around the belly, thighs and hips), which ultimately results to fat loss and subsequent weight loss.

✓ Additionally, intermittent fasting triggers your body's metabolism rate through the human growth hormone (HGH). When you fast, the body responds by releasing more HGH, a fat burning hormone that helps maintain your muscle mass while fasting. A higher metabolism rate means that your body gets to use up calories fast and this leads to weight loss without losing muscle mass.

✓ In addition, intermittent fasting can help you combat your hunger and cravings, which often push you to snack unnecessarily and ultimately make you to have caloric surpluses. With reduced cravings and hunger cravings, you end up eating less, which means that creating the much needed caloric deficit for weight loss becomes pretty easy. So why does that happen? Well, IF helps to normalize or reduce ghrelin (the hunger hormone). This ultimately helps give you less appetite.

So these are the ways intermittent fasting helps to hasten short term and long term weight loss. In fact some people have confirmed that they lost up to 5 to 8 pounds a week by engaging in intermittent fasting.

It Helps To Boost Your Body's Immune System

Your immune system is the part of your body that helps to fight against germs, antibodies and micro organisms that cause sickness. When there is a boost in your immune system, it means that your body can actively fight and kick out any disease causing microorganism within your body. One way to boost your body's immunity level is through intermittent fasting. During the fast, your body tries to conserve energy and one way it does that is to recycle weak or damaged immune cells for your body to produce new immune cells- the immune cells can be damaged by chemotherapy or aging process. Intermittent fasting helps to recycle the damaged cells to produce new cells. This helps to prevent diseases such as Alzheimer's and cancer, and slows down the aging process. In addition, intermittent fasting helps to trigger autophagy, which is a process of cellular repair in which waste is eliminated from the body cells.

It Helps Reduce Cholesterol Level

High level of cholesterol in the blood is one of the factors that trigger many heart related diseases. As the body uses up fats, the LDL cholesterol level is reduced considerably, and it is not just cholesterol that is affected by this process; the blood pressure and blood triglycerides are also reduced considerably. That's why it is safe to say that intermittent fasting helps to reduce the chances of developing heart diseases.

It Helps To Prevent Insulin Resistance

Insulin resistance is one of the major causes of the Type 2 diabetes. Insulin resistance occurs when your body cannot effectively make use of the insulin produced or when the body cannot produce enough insulin to keep up with the demand for insulin in the body. The resultant effect is that the body cells are not triggered to absorb sugar from the blood, and a buildup of glucose in the blood stream is what causes the Type 2 diabetes (this happens when there is consistently high level of blood glucose. Intermittent fasting helps to prevent and reverse insulin resistance. When you go on intermittent fasting, it helps to reduce and reverse insulin resistance because when the body is in a fasting mode, it is forced to absorb glucose from the blood stream to produce energy before it can even start using up stored glycogen and subsequently stored fat. Ultimately, intermittent fasting increases insulin sensitivity and causes a reduction in the mitochondrial energy. With improved insulin sensitivity, this means that your body will require small amounts of insulin to lower your blood sugar level because your body cells are highly sensitive to signals from insulin to absorb sugar from the blood. Research has shown that people with Type 2 diabetes were able to normalize their blood sugar levels after few weeks of intermittent fasting.

It Helps To Reduce Oxidative Stress

Oxidative stress occurs when the bad molecules in your body, which are often known as free radicals, damage good molecules such as DNA and proteins. Intermittent fasting helps your body to develop resistance to oxidative stress and fight against inflammation in the body. It does this by reducing the accumulation of oxidative radicals in your body cells. This process prevents the oxidative damage of good molecules like lipid, cellular proteins and nucleic acid.

It Helps To Kill Of Cancerous Cells

One of the common diseases making waves in the world today is cancer. Millions of people die from complications related to cancer every single year. The good news is that intermittent fasting can help prevent and cure cancer. Cancer occurs when body cells begin to multiply in an uncontrollable number. One thing about cancerous cells is that they feed on glucose or blood sugar. When there is enough glucose in the blood, cancerous cells are sustained and continue with the robotic growth. But the good news is that fasting actually creates a hostile environment for the cancerous cells. When you are fasting, your blood sugar level drops considerably because the body uses up all the glucose in the bloodstream and has to rely on the liver to create ketone bodies from the liver. Ketone bodies are an alternative source of energy that the body relies on when you are on prolonged fasting. The resultant effect is that there won't be enough glucose for the cancerous cell to feed on thus they start to die off. This same process works with precancerous cells i.e. cells that cause cancer. It has even been confirmed that intermittent fasting is a more effective remedy for cancer than chemotherapy.

It Makes You Feel Good

Besides the fact that weight loss because of fasting helps you feel good about yourself and boosts your self-esteem, intermittent fating is known to release a higher level of endorphins in your body. The endorphin is that hormone that makes you feel good. Secondly, it increases your brain derived neurotrophic factor, and the absence of this BDNF can lead to depression and other brain complications.

Obviously, these are not all the benefits that come with intermittent fasting. You can derive many more benefits from intermittent fasting. You can read more about that here. But even with all these benefits, intermittent fasting, just like anything else in life, comes with its own set of challenges or risks that you need to be aware of. Let's discuss some of these risks in the next chapter.

Health Risks Associated with Intermittent Fasting

With all these benefits mentioned above, you may want to know if there are any health risks associated with intermittent fasting. The truth is that there are some minor health risks associated to fasting, and it is beneficial to mention those risks in order to give you a holistic view of what intermittent fasting entails. Some of the risks associated with fasting include:

a. **Dehydration**

Most people have little or no urge to drink water when they are fasting because they say that it helps to reduce the hunger pangs. On the contrary, the truth is that this exposes them to the risk of dehydration since they are not taking in any fluid from either water or food. This is because during intermittent fasting, your body continues to lose water and salt through urinating, perspiration and breathing. When you don't intake enough water to replenish the water and salt lost, it can lead to dehydration. Some of the health complications associated with dehydration are; dry skin, dizziness, rapid heartbeat, low blood pressure, headache, irritability, and extreme thirst. The solution to this is to ensure that you drink plenty water during your fasting period. Besides, for you to lose weight sustainably, your body processes (metabolism) will need water to function at optimal capacity. That's why you will need to drink water regularly for you to derive the various benefits that come with IF. In fact, taking water can help make you feel full without increasing your calorie intake (water has zero calories). But if you don't like the taste of plain water, you may want to add some lemon to your water to make it tastier.

b. **Increase In Stress Level**

When there is a sudden interruption in your regular eating schedule, it can lead to stress. For instance, if you are used to eating breakfast once you wake up, when you go on intermittent fasting pattern that will require you to skip breakfast, your body may enter a stress mode. This is because intermittent fasting triggers the release of hormones like cortisol and adrenalin, the stress hormones. Cortisol is secreted in the adrenal gland and is affected by the level of glucose in your bloodstream. When there is a calorie deficit in your body as a result of fasting, your blood sugar level is reduced and this in turn triggers the release of cortisol. The more cortisol that is released, the more stressed you will feel. This can disrupt your sleep cycle and probably affect your ability to derive the most benefits from IF. That's why you will need to tailor your intermittent fasting schedule in a way that enables you to fast without putting too much strain on your eating schedule. For instance, you can work towards making your sleeping hours part of your 'fasting' hours in order to reduce the number of fasted hours that you are awake.

c. **It Causes Heartburn**

Whenever you eat, your body produces a stomach acid that helps to break down the food for digestion. When you are fasting, the level of stomach acid is reduced to the barest minimum. But when you start thinking of food or you perceive the smell of food, your brain will send a signal to your stomach to start production of stomach acids. When the stomach acid is produced and there is no food to break down, it will result to heartburn. Heartburn can be relieved with an antacid tablet but you can make use any of the following remedies:

- Baking soda as it serves as a quick relief for heartburn. Get half a teaspoon of baking soda, mix in one cup of water and drink. Baking soda or sodium bicarbonate contains a high Ph level which is above 7.0. Thus, it helps to neutralize the stomach acid.

- Aloe vera: Aloe vera helps to reduce inflammation in the body and provides a soothing effect. Drink a cup of aloe gel for fast relief.

- Chewing gum is another remedy for heartburn. Chewing gum stimulates your salivary glands to release more saliva. The increase in the flow of saliva washes away any acid that is built up in your gut and provides relief for heartburn. A stick of sugar-free gum can provide relief for heartburn in as little as 30 minutes.

d. **It is Not Recommended For Everybody**

Unlike other diets or eating lifestyles that can be incorporated by everybody, intermittent fasting is not good for everybody. In particular, you should not go on intermittent fasting if you:

Suffer from type 1 diabetes: For persons with the Type 1 diabetes especially when you take regular insulin injections, IF can be very harmful to your health. Intermittent fasting causes your blood glucose level to drop and the role of insulin injection is to reduce your blood glucose level. The effect is that it causes your blood glucose level to drop lower than the normal level. This is called hypoglycaemia and is a very serious health condition. In addition, intermittent fasting can also trigger a condition known as hyperglycemia, which makes your blood sugar to rise above the normal level because of buildup of ketones, which leads to a health condition known as ketoacidosis. Thus, if you have type 1 diabetes, it is advisable not to go on IF unless you are closely monitored to accurately keep track of your blood sugar level and to reduce your dose of insulin injections.

Are underweight: For an underweight person, intermittent fasting can lead to malnutrition as the body will be forced to stay without adequate diet and will also be forced to give up the little fats that are stored up.

Are pregnant: Pregnant women are advised to stay away from any form of fasting because it can lead to premature labor. IF can also cause a low birth weight and in most cases, it can deprive the unborn child of some vital nutrients, which would be derived from food.

e. It Can Trigger Eating Disorders

Some dieticians have advised that intermittent fasting or prolonged fasting can trigger eating disorders such as binge eating disorder. Although this is yet to not be confirmed, some scientists assume there is link between intermittent fasting and eating disorders especially binge eating. Some researchers are of the view that long abstinence from food can trigger the release of ghrelin, which is the hormone that is responsible for hunger.

f. It Is Not Ideal For Long Term Weight Loss

Some fitness experts are of the view that intermittent fasting is not ideal for long-term weight loss. To them, if the fats can come off quickly, they can also come back quickly. They are of the view that intermittent fasting should not be used as a long term weight loss goal because once you revert back to your normal eating style, you can still regain the lost weight. This is not necessarily true because intermittent fasting should not be seen as a quick fix for weight loss but as a lifestyle. Also, strength training during intermittent fasting helps to keep the fats off for good.

Now that you have a good understanding of what IF is all about as well as some of the risks that come with intermittent fasting, I know you are excited to start your journey to losing weight and deriving all the benefits that we've already discussed about. As we stated, IF is all about when you eat than what you eat so how do you optimize your 'when you eat' time to derive the most benefits from IF? We will discuss some eating patterns in the next chapter.

Types Of Intermittent Fasting

At this stage, you now know the meaning of intermittent fasting; the health benefits that you stand to gain from practicing intermittent fasting and some of the challenges/problems of the fasting. This section will focus on discussing the types or methods of intermittent fasting or simply the eating patterns that you can follow. There are basically five popular types of intermittent fasting. Which of these five types of intermittent fasting is best for me? You are in a better position to answer that question because the type of intermittent fasting you incorporate will be dependent on several factors such as the type of job your do and the amount of weight you want to lose. I will discuss these five types of fasting in detail and for each I mention, I will include the pros and cons. This will help you make a better choice on the type of fasting that will suit your daily needs.

The Lean Gain Intermittent Fasting

Martin Berkhan popularized this type of intermittent fasting. It requires you to fast for at least 14 to 16 hours every single day.

If you are a male, you are required to fast for at least 16 hours every day. This leaves you with an eight hours window period (feeding time) daily. You can eat your normal meals within the eight hours but fasting commences after the end of the window period. A typical time frame for a lean-gain fasting is to start your fasting around 6pm everyday. Then your window period starts by 10am the following morning and ends by 5 pm. During this period, you are allowed to eat your normal meals for the day in moderate proportions.

If you are a female on the other hand, this type of intermittent fasting allows you to fast for 14 hours and gives you a 10 hours window period everyday. Therefore, your typical day of fasting will start from 8pm and end 10am the following morning while your window period starts from 10am and ends by 7 pm.

It is very easy to lose weight fast with this type of fasting as you fast everyday. When I tried to experiment with this type of fasting, I actually lost 3 pounds within a week, may be because I restricted my calorie intake for the week to just 1,000 for each day.

Pros Of The Lean-Gain Fasting

- The first is that this type of fast is newbie friendly so a newbie can easily start with this type of fasting. Eating dinner at 6pm and breakfast around 10am will not be hard to maintain for a newbie. Therefore, I will advise you to start with this type of fasting if this is your first time fasting.

- You can incorporate a three square meal within your 8-10 hours window period. Your body won't feel deprived when you do so.

The 5:2 Fasting Diet

Dr. Michael Mosley popularized this type of intermittent fasting. For this type of fast, you are to eat your normal calorie requirement for 5 days a week. The normal calorie requirement for men is 2,500 kcal daily and 2,000kcal for women.

Choose two days in a week when you will fast. For the days you will fast, you will be required to eat just 500 calories if you are a woman and 600 calories if you are a man. So how do you implement this eating pattern? Well, you can eat your normal calorie intake on Monday,

Wednesday, Friday, Saturday and Sunday. Then on Tuesday and Thursday, you eat two meals of 250 calories each. This type of fasting is known to aid weight loss without strenuous activities.

Pros Of The 5:2 Fasting Diet

- You get to lose weight eating whatever you want as long as it is within the calorie limit on none fasting (feeding) days because your body will use up the extra calories on the days you fast.

Important note about the 5: 2 fast

- You need to be conscious of your calorie intake on your fasting days to ensure that you don't eat above the permitted limit.

- There is a need to stay away from very strenuous activities during your fasting days. In essence, if you are a sportsman, then this type of fasting is not for you.

-

The Eat Stop Eat Fasting

Brad Pilon popularized this type of fasting. This type of fasting is almost similar to the one discussed above, but it is still different in its own way. For 'the eat stop eat fasting', you eat your normal meals for 5 days in a week, then you choose two days of your choice to fast. The unique thing about this type of fasting is that on your fasting days, you are not required to eat any form of solid food. It has to be an absolute fasting, but you are permitted to drink water and any other drink with no calorie content like lime or lemon water and coffee without sugar or cream.

Tip: This type of fasting is best for people who have reached a plateau in their weight loss journey. There comes a time in your weight loss journey when it seems that your body has stopped losing weight no matter the efforts you make. The eat stop eat fasting can trigger your body to break down the stubborn fats to enable you reach your ideal weight.

Pros Of The Eat Stop Eat Fasting Method

- This type of fasting comes in handy when you have reached your weight loss plateau. Staying 24 hours without food turns your body into a fat burning machine. The good thing is that your body uses fats only even after 24 hours of fasting.

The Cons Of The Eat Stop Eat Fasting Method

- It is difficult for a newbie to adapt to this type of fasting. Imagine telling someone who rarely skips breakfast to embark on a 24 hours fasting regime. The answer you will get from the person will certainly be a negative answer. Therefore, this type of fasting is not ideal for a newbie.

- Also, this form of fasting is not ideal for you especially if you engage in strenuous activities for long hours at a time.

- This type of fasting is likely to trigger binge eating. Staying for 24 hours without eating may trigger a huge release of the ghrelin hormone, which is responsible for hunger pangs. If you don't have the self-discipline to eat moderately, you can give in to binge eating.

-

The Alternate Day Fasting

This method of fasting requires that you alternate your fasting days. It means that you have to fast every other day. This method of fasting is also similar to the 5:2 days fasting method but requires that you fast every other day and not just twice a week. An example of how this type of fasting can be implemented is: you eat your normal calorie of 2,000 kcal today, then the next day, you just eat 500 calories. The day after the next, you revert back to 2,000 kcal. You continue to alternate your fasting days until you achieve your desired weight loss goals.

Pros Of The alternate Day Fasting Method

- It is newbie friendly because a newbie can endure a 500 kcal day knowing that he will eat his normal calorie requirement the next day.

Cons Of The Alternate Fasting

- There is a need to keep track of calories especially on days you fast.

- The alternation between eating your normal calorie and fewer calorie days can trigger cortisol, which is the stress causing hormone.

Warrior Diet

This type of fasting, as the name implies, is not for the faint hearted. This type of fasting requires that you maintain a fasting period of over 20 hours every day. This leaves you with a 4 hours window period. The person that popularized the warrior diet is called Ori Hofmekler. This method of fasting requires strict discipline to follow through. You are required to eat one heavy meal at night just before you sleep but you are permitted to eat several servings of raw fruits and vegetables throughout the day. You have to be mindful of the content of your large meal at night because the meal should be well balanced to provide your body with the nutrients and energy required to function the next day. The meal should contain more of lean proteins and fiber (from vegetable).

Pros Of The Warrior Diet

- It helps to maximize nutrients use. Your digestive system is free from work all day during the warrior fast period. This makes it work actively to absorb all the nutrients needed for growth and tissue repairs from that single meal.

- It helps in extreme weight loss as your body is turned into a fat burning machine during the day.

- It helps to optimize the activity of parasympathetic nerves, which helps your body to recuperate.

Cons Of The Warrior Diet

- Staying for almost 24 hours without food may trigger binge eating disorder if you lack the self-discipline to control your appetite.

- This type of fasting is not newbie friendly.

From all the above intermittent eating patterns, I know you are asking; ***What Type Of Fasting Best Fits Me***?

I mentioned earlier that the method of intermittent fasting you adopt depends on several factors. I have discussed the various methods of engaging in intermittent fasting with the pros and cons of each method. If your main goal is to lose weight fast and build muscles and you have the self-discipline to control your appetite, I will advise you to go for the warrior fasting or eat stop eat fasting. But if on the other hand you are a newbie and you want to try out this intermittent fasting without subjecting yourself to much stress, you can go for either the lean gain, the alternate fasting or the 5: 2 days fasting methods.

To help you throughout the journey to losing weight and obtaining various other benefits, let's now discuss some tips and tricks that can help you make IF more effective.

Tips To Make Your Fasting More Effective

There are some things you can do to make your intermittent fast more effective. They include:

- **Start Up Small**

Starting up with the Warrior or the 24 hours fasting when you can barely complete the lean-gain fast is one recipe for failure. For you to successfully incorporate the intermittent fasting as a lifestyle, it is advisable that you start small. You can begin with a 12 hours fasting for one week; when your body gets used to the process, you can add another one or two hours to it. This also helps to reduce the level of cortisol that is released in your body, thus subjecting your body to very little stress.

- **Fruits and Vegetables Are Allowed**

Although you are likely to get the best result from intermittent fasting by taking only water during your fasting period, you are advised to eat several servings of fruits and vegetables through the fast to help keep the hunger pangs away. Fruits in this context include fruits with very little calorie content such as apple, watermelon or cucumber. Avoid fruits like avocado, pears and banana during the fasting period because they contain lots of calories. In addition, vegetables should include just green leafy vegetables and other types of vegetables, which can be eaten raw for instance carrot. Fruits and vegetables will provide your body with the minimal energy needed to keep up with your daily activities. Also, it will keep you full, which is necessary to avoid binge eating your first meal after fasting.

- Allow Your Fasting Encroach Into The Night

As you schedule a timeframe for your fasting, try to ensure that it encroaches into the night. You will likely not feel the hunger pangs when you are asleep.

- Moderation Is The Key

You can optimize the effects of you fasting by the way and what you eat after your fast. Your first meal after fasting is very essential and you need to ensure that first, you eat in a moderate quantity and secondly that the meal contains just the essential nutrients needed by the body. Taking fruits and vegetables throughout the day will help you maintain moderation for your first meal. Secondly, the meal should be made up of lean proteins, loaded with vegetables, and a smaller amount of carbohydrates and fats. Avoid processed carbohydrates or sugar as much as you can because they provide your body with little or no nutrients.

- Exercise

If you want to lose weight faster, then you need to include some form of physical exercise into your intermittent fasting schedule. Remember that fasting turns your body into a fat burning machine. If you include physical exercise, especially aerobic exercises, which helps to speed up your heartbeat, you will burn fats at a faster rate.

If you cannot withstand aerobic exercises during your fasting period, then you can stick to strength training or weight lifting because it will still help you achieve the same result. Strength training helps to build your muscles since fats are used as you build muscles. To get maximum results, you should schedule your workout time to be two hours before you end your fast. For instance, if your window period is to commence by 11am, you can schedule a workout for 9am.

Conclusion

Thank you again for downloading this book!

I hope this book was able to help you to understand how to use intermittent fasting for a wide array of benefits.

The next step is to use what you have learnt to obtain some of the benefits you've learnt.

Finally, if you enjoyed this book, would you be kind enough to leave a review for this book on Amazon?

Click here to leave a review for this book on Amazon!

Thank you and good luck!